The Ultimate Plant-Based Diet Cookbook

Discover Fabulous Plant-Based Recipes to Create Tasty and Healthy Dishes

By
Candace Dawson

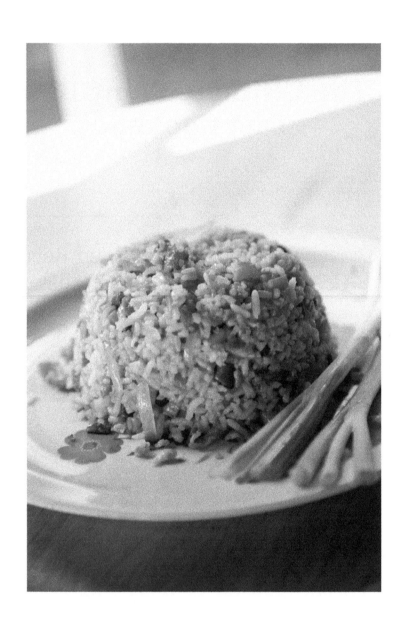

the publisher or the original author of this work can be in any fashion deemed liable for any hardship or damages that may befall them after undertaking information described herein.

Additionally, the information in the following pages is intended only for informational purposes and should thus be thought of as universal. As befitting its nature, it is presented without assurance regarding its prolonged validity or interim quality. Trademarks that are mentioned are done without written consent and can in no way be considered an endorsement from the trademark holder.

Table of Contents

6

Desserts 89

Introduction

What is the Plant Based Diet?

The Plant Based diet is mostly a plant-based diet. Was born from a conviction that food is medicine. This diet focuses on the nature of the foods he eats. Researchers support a move away from factory production and refined foods. Instead, he emphasizes whole foods from plants, healthy fats, and grass fed proteins in his diet. Continue reading to learn more about the Plant Based Diet.

Principles of a Plant Based Diet

Omega-3 fats (fatty fish and flaxseeds) are recommended, as well as fats from nuts, seeds, coconut, and avocados. About Pegan recipes, the consumption of saturated fats from grass-fed or sustainably raised livestock, but only in limited quantities.

Vegetable oils, eggs, gluten, and grains are not used in this recipe. Sugar consumption in any form is discouraged. Legume consumption is limited. Pesticides, antibiotics, hormones, and GMOs can all be stopped by consuming organic foods.

Potential Health Implications of the Plant Based Diet

Several principles of the Plant Based diet are decided upon by nutrition experts. For instance, they agree that having fruits, vegetables, and omega-3 fats in one's diet is beneficial to one's health and weight loss. These foods also aid in nutrient absorption and cancer and disease prevention. Second, they accept that sugar and meat intake should be very reduced. This aids in the prevention of heart disease and diabetes.

On the other hand, nutritionists disagree with excluding and limiting food classes unless there is a genuine allergy or intolerance. Food restriction can cause an insufficient intake of nutrients that can help improve health outcomes. The Plant Based Diet, for example, doesn't limit the intake of whole grains, according to nutritionists' guidelines. Consumption of whole grains is related to a lower risk of cardiovascular disease and blood glucose levels. They, along with legumes, are also high in dietary fiber, which can help minimize the risk of cancer, diabetes, and other health problems.

The plant-based diet meets conventional dietary guidelines, however an approach is suggested in this book to minimally integrate foods excluded from the conventional plant-based diet, for this reason some recipes of the Pegan diet are included. However, consult your healthcare professional before starting any diet. This will help you avoid nutrient deficiencies and find a program that is personalized to your individual health needs.

Benefits of the Plant Based Diet

The Plant Based diet emphasizes whole foods rich in vitamins and minerals your body needs. This will result in substantial weight loss on the Plant Based diet, depending on your current diet.

For someone who consumes a conventional Western diet high in refined foods, the benefits of the Plant Based diet can be much more apparent than for someone who already eats a balanced diet.

Furthermore, the diet emphasizes nutritious foods that can help boost a variety of facets of wellness, including heart health, blood sugar levels, and disease prevention, in addition to weight loss. Healthy oils, fruits, vegetables, some of the healthiest nuts, seeds, and renewable protein sources are all included in the Plant Based diet, and they can all be perfect additions to a well-rounded diet.

Breakfast

Maca Caramel Frap

Preparation time: 5 minutes
Cooking time: 0 minute
Servings: 4

Ingredients:
- 1/2 of frozen banana, sliced
- 1/4 cup cashews, soaked for 4 hours
- 2 Medjool dates, pitted
- 1 teaspoon maca powder
- 1/8 teaspoon sea salt
- 1/2 teaspoon vanilla extract, unsweetened
- 1/4 cup almond milk, unsweetened
- 1/4 cup cold coffee, brewed

Directions:
1. Place all the ingredients in the order in a food processor or blender and then pulse for 2 to 3 minutes at high speed until smooth.
2. Pour the smoothie into a glass and then serve.

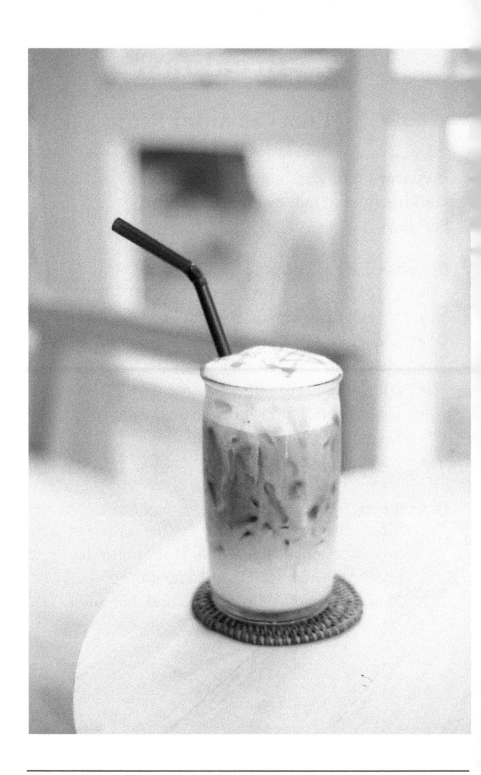

Green Colada

Preparation time: 5 minutes
Cooking time: 0 minute
Servings: 1

Ingredients:
- 1/2 cup frozen pineapple chunks
- 1/2 banana
- 1/2 teaspoon spirulina powder
- 1/4 teaspoon vanilla extract, unsweetened
- 1 cup of coconut milk

Directions:
1. Place all the ingredients in the order in a food processor or blender and then pulse for 2 to 3 minutes at high speed until smooth.
2. Pour the smoothie into a glass and then serve.

Peach Crumble Shake

Preparation time: 5 minutes
Cooking time: 0 minute
Servings: 1

Ingredients:
- 1 tablespoon chia seeds
- ¼ cup rolled oats
- 2 peaches, pitted, sliced
- ¾ teaspoon ground cinnamon
- 1 Medjool date, pitted
- ½ teaspoon vanilla extract, unsweetened
- 2 tablespoons lemon juice
- ½ cup of water
- 1 tablespoon coconut butter
- 1 cup coconut milk, unsweetened

Directions:
1. Place all the ingredients in the order in a food processor or blender and then pulse for 2 to 3 minutes at high speed until smooth.
2. Pour the smoothie into a glass and then serve.

Berry Beet Velvet Smoothie

Preparation time: 5 minutes
Cooking time: 0 minute
Servings: 1

Ingredients:
- 1/2 of frozen banana
- 1 cup mixed red berries
- 1 Medjool date, pitted
- 1 small beet, peeled, chopped
- 1 tablespoon cacao powder
- 1 teaspoon chia seeds
- 1/4 teaspoon vanilla extract, unsweetened
- 1/2 teaspoon lemon juice
- 2 teaspoons coconut butter
- 1 cup coconut milk, unsweetened

Directions:
1. Place all the ingredients in the order in a food processor or blender and then pulse for 2 to 3 minutes at high speed until smooth.
2. Pour the smoothie into a glass and then serve.

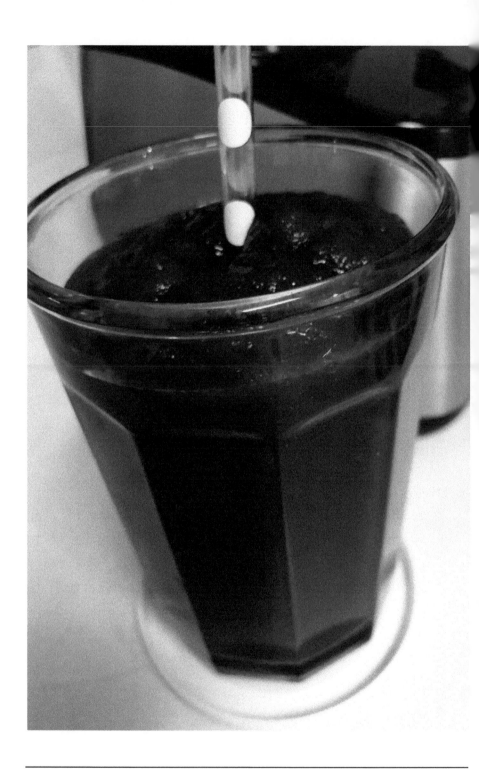

Banana Bread Shake With Walnut Milk

Preparation time: 5 minutes
Cooking time: 0 minute
Servings: 2

Ingredients:
- 2 cups sliced frozen bananas
- 3 cups walnut milk
- 1/8 teaspoon grated nutmeg
- 1 tablespoon maple syrup
- 1 teaspoon ground cinnamon
- 1/2 teaspoon vanilla extract, unsweetened
- 2 tablespoons cacao nibs

Directions:
1. Place all the ingredients in the order in a food processor or blender and then pulse for 2 to 3 minutes at high speed until smooth.
2. Pour the smoothie into two glasses and then serve.

Strawberry, Banana and Coconut Shake

Preparation time: 5 minutes
Cooking time: 0 minute
Servings: 1

Ingredients:
- 1 tablespoon coconut flakes
- 1 1/2 cups frozen banana slices
- 8 strawberries, sliced
- 1/2 cup coconut milk, unsweetened
- 1/4 cup strawberries for topping

Directions:
1. Place all the ingredients in the order in a food processor or blender, except for topping and then pulse for 2 to 3 minutes at high speed until smooth.
2. Pour the smoothie into a glass and then serve.

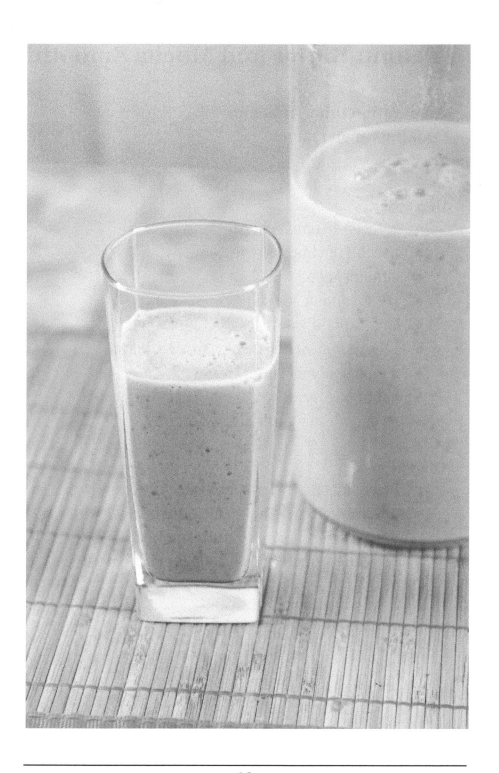

Peanut Butter and Mocha Smoothie

Preparation time: 5 minutes
Cooking time: 0 minute
Servings: 1

Ingredients:
- 1 frozen banana, chopped
- 1 scoop of chocolate protein powder
- 2 tablespoons rolled oats
- 1/8 teaspoon sea salt
- ¼ teaspoon vanilla extract, unsweetened
- 1 teaspoon cocoa powder, unsweetened
- 2 tablespoons peanut butter
- 1 shot of espresso
- ½ cup almond milk, unsweetened

Directions:
1. Place all the ingredients in the order in a food processor or blender and then pulse for 2 to 3 minutes at high speed until smooth.
2. Pour the smoothie into a glass and then serve.

Ginger and Greens Smoothie

Preparation time: 5 minutes
Cooking time: 0 minute
Servings: 1

Ingredients:
- 1 frozen banana
- 2 cups baby spinach
- 2-inch piece of ginger, peeled, chopped
- ¼ teaspoon cinnamon
- ¼ teaspoon vanilla extract, unsweetened
- 1/8 teaspoon salt
- 1 scoop vanilla protein powder
- 1/8 teaspoon cayenne pepper
- 2 tablespoons lemon juice
- 1 cup of orange juice

Directions:
1. Place all the ingredients in the order in a food processor or blender and then pulse for 2 to 3 minutes at high speed until smooth.
2. Pour the smoothie into a glass and then serve.

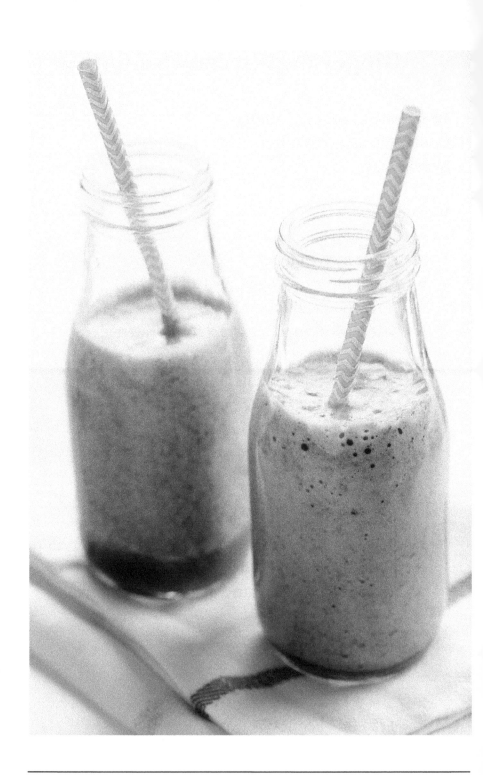

Sweet Potato Smoothie

Preparation time: 5 minutes
Cooking time: 0 minute
Servings: 1

Ingredients:
- 1/2 cup frozen zucchini pieces
- 1 cup cubed cooked sweet potato, frozen
- 1/2 frozen banana
- 1/2 teaspoon sea salt
- 1/2 teaspoon cinnamon
- 1 scoop of vanilla protein powder
- 1/4 teaspoon nutmeg
- 1 tablespoon almond butter
- 1 1/2 cups almond milk, unsweetened

Directions:
1. Place all the ingredients in the order in a food processor or blender and then pulse for 2 to 3 minutes at high speed until smooth.
2. Pour the smoothie into a glass and then serve.

Chocolate Cherry Smoothie

Preparation time: 5 minutes
Cooking time: 0 minute
Servings: 1

Ingredients:
- 1 1/2 cups frozen cherries, pitted
- 1 cup spinach
- 1/2 small frozen banana
- 2 tablespoon cacao powder, unsweetened
- 1 tablespoon chia seeds
- 1 scoop of vanilla protein powder
- 1 teaspoon spirulina
- 1 1/2 cups almond milk, unsweetened

Directions:
1. Place all the ingredients in the order in a food processor or blender and then pulse for 2 to 3 minutes at high speed until smooth.
2. Pour the smoothie into a glass and then serve.

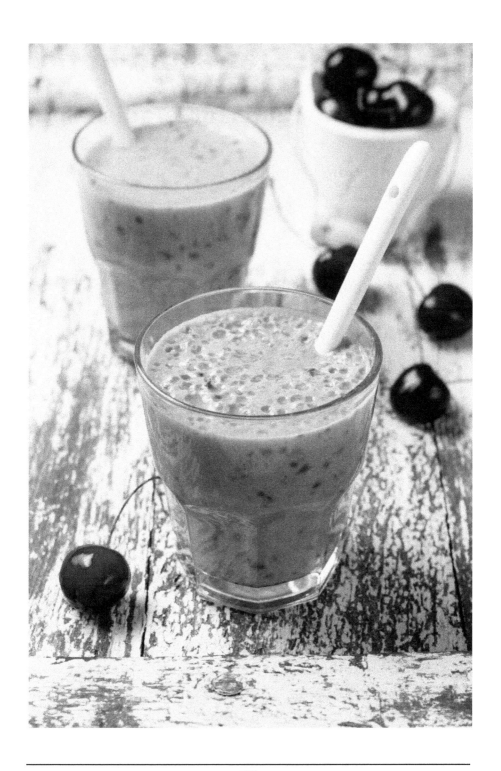

Soups, Stews and Lunch

Cauliflower and Horseradish Soup

Preparation time: 5 minutes
Cooking time: 20 minutes
Servings: 4

Ingredients:
- 2 medium potatoes, peeled, chopped
- 1 medium cauliflower, florets and stalk chopped
- 1 medium white onion, peeled, chopped
- 1 teaspoon minced garlic
- 2/3 teaspoon salt
- 1/3 teaspoon ground black pepper
- 4 teaspoons horseradish sauce
- 1 teaspoon dried thyme
- 3 cups vegetable broth
- 1 cup coconut milk, unsweetened

Directions:
1. Place all the vegetables in a large pan, place it over medium-high heat, add thyme, pour in broth and milk and bring the mixture to boil.
2. Then switch heat to medium level, simmer the soup for 15 minutes and remove the pan from heat.
3. Puree the soup by using an immersion blender until smooth, season with salt and black pepper, and serve straight away.

Chickpea Noodle Soup

Preparation time: 5 minutes
Cooking time: 18 minutes
Servings: 6

Ingredients:
- 1 cup cooked chickpeas
- 8 ounces rotini noodles, whole-wheat
- 4 celery stalks, sliced
- 2 medium white onions, peeled, chopped
- 4 medium carrots, peeled, sliced
- 2 teaspoons minced garlic
- 8 sprigs of thyme
- 1 teaspoon salt
- 1/3 teaspoon ground black pepper
- 1 bay leaf
- 2 tablespoons olive oil
- 2 quarts of vegetable broth
- ¼ cup chopped fresh parsley

Directions:
1. Take a large pot, place it over medium heat, add oil and when hot, add all the vegetables, stir in garlic, thyme and bay leaf and cook for 5 minutes until vegetables are golden and sauté.
2. Then pour in broth, stir and bring the mixture to boil.
3. Add chickpeas and noodles into boiling soup, continue cooking for 8 minutes until noodles are

tender, and then season soup with salt and black pepper.

4. Garnish with parsley and serve straight away

Quinoa Pepper Burgers

Preparation time: 10 minutes
Cooking time: 30 minutes
Servings: 6–8 burgers

Ingredients:
- 2/3 cup uncooked quinoa
- 3 cups water or vegetable broth
- 4 roasted red bell peppers
- 1 cup canned white beans
- 2 tablespoons chopped coriander
- Salt, pepper (to taste)

Directions:
1. Bring 3 cups of water/broth to a boil.
2. Add quinoa, remove from heat and allow quinoa to absorb all of the liquid.
3. Combine the bell pepper and beans in a food processor and pulse until a paste forms.
4. In a medium mixing bowl, combine paste, quinoa, coriander, and salt/pepper.
5. Using wet hands, form the mixture into a burger shape.
6. Add one tablespoon of olive oil to the frying pan and heat over medium.
7. Cook burgers on each side for 7 minutes, until crispy.

Tropical Island Burgers

Preparation time: 10 minutes
Cooking time: 30 minutes
Servings: 6–8 burgers

Ingredients:
- 3 cups canned black beans, rinsed and drained
- 1/2 cup rolled oats
- 4 tablespoons sweet corn
- 1/4 cup crushed pineapple
- 1 teaspoon mustard
- Salt, pepper (to taste)

Directions:
1. Create a paste with beans and oats by pulsing in the food processor.
2. In a large mixing bowl, combine paste with the remaining ingredient list.
3. Using wet hands, form the mixture into a burger shape.
4. Add one tablespoon of olive oil to the frying pan and heat over medium.
5. Cook burgers on each side for 7 minutes, until brown and crispy.

Fennel and Beetroot Burger

Preparation time: 10 minutes
Cooking time: 50 minutes
Servings: 6–8 burgers

Ingredients:
- 2 medium size beetroots, peeled and grated
- 2 tablespoons chopped dill
- 1 fennel bulb, trimmed and finely chopped
- 1 cup cooked brown rice
- 2 tablespoons cornmeal
- 1/4 cup tomato sauce
- Salt, pepper (tp taste)

Directions:
1. In a large mixing bowl, combine grated beets, fennel, dill, brown rice and cornmeal.
2. Stir in the tomato sauce, salt/pepper, and form small patties.
3. Add one tablespoon of olive oil to the frying pan and fry the burger for 6 minutes on each side.
4. Serve on vegan burger buns and favorite toppings

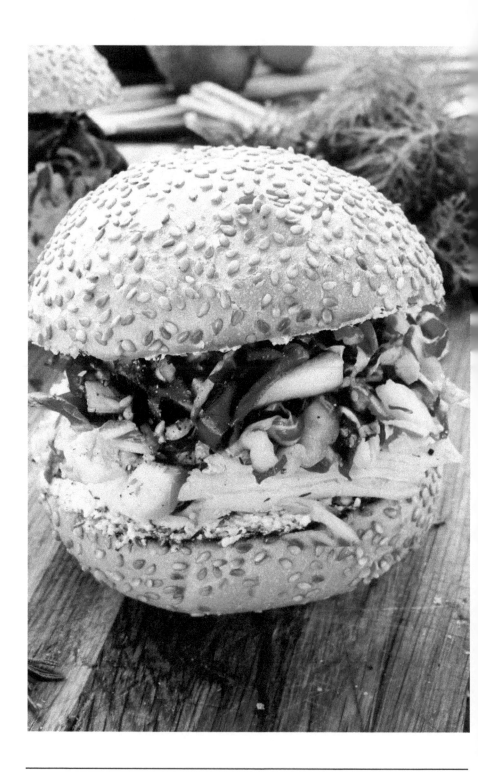

Sautéed Green Beans, Mushrooms & Tomatoes

Preparation Time: 15 minutes
Cooking Time: 15 minutes
Servings: 10

Ingredients:

- Water 3 lb. green beans, trimmed
- 2 tablespoons olive oil
- 8 cloves garlic, minced
- ½ cup tomato, diced
- 12 oz. cremini mushrooms, sliced into quarters
- Salt and pepper to taste

Directions:

1. Fill a pot with water.
2. Bring to a boil.
3. Add the beans and cook for 5 minutes.
4. Drain the beans.
5. Dry the pot.
6. Pour oil into the pot.
7. Add garlic, tomato and mushrooms.
8. Cook for 5 minutes.
9. Add the beans and cook for another 5 minutes.
10. Season with salt and pepper.
11. Store in a food container and reheat before eating.

Green Beans, Roasted Red Peppers & Onions

Preparation Time: 15 minutes
Cooking Time: 25 minutes
Servings: 6

Ingredients:
- 1 tablespoon olive oil
- 1 ½ cups onion, chopped
- 1 tablespoon red wine vinegar
- ½ cup jarred roasted red peppers, drained and chopped
- 2 tablespoons fresh basil, chopped
- ¼ cup olives, pitted and sliced
- Salt and pepper to taste
- 1 lb. fresh green beans, trimmed and sliced

Directions:
1. Pour olive oil in a pan over medium heat.
2. Add onion and cook for 10 minutes.
3. Pour in the vinegar.
4. Cook for 2 minutes.
5. Add roasted red peppers, basil and olives.
6. Season with salt and pepper.
7. Remove from the stove.
8. In a saucepan with water, cook beans for 10 minutes.
9. Add beans to the onion mixture.
10. Stir for 3 minutes.

Sweet Spicy Beans

Preparation Time: 10 minutes
Cooking Time: 50 minutes
Servings: 10

Ingredients:
- 3 tablespoons vegetable oil
- 1 onion, chopped
- 45 oz. navy beans, rinsed and drained
- 1 ½ cups water
- ¾ cup ketchup
- 1/3 cup brown sugar
- 1 tablespoon white vinegar
- 1 teaspoon chipotle peppers in adobo sauce
- Salt and pepper to taste

Directions:
1. Pour the oil in a pan over medium heat.
2. Add onion and cook for 10 minutes.
3. Add the rest of the Ingredients.
4. Bring to a boil.
5. Reduce heat and simmer for 30 minutes.
6. Transfer to a food container.
7. Reheat when ready to eat.

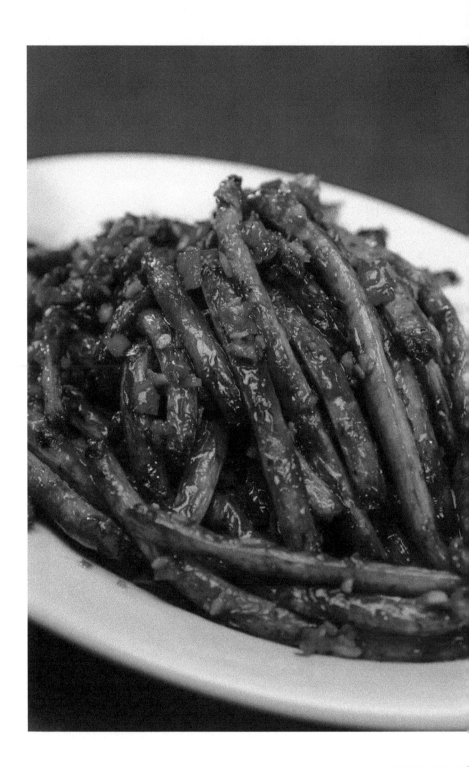

Creamy Veggie Risotto

Preparation time: 15 minutes
Cooking time: 35 minutes
Servings: 4

Ingredients:
- 2 Tablespoons Olive Oil
- 1 Clove Garlic, Minced
- ½ Sweet Onion, Diced
- 1 Bunch Asparagus Tips, Chopped into 1 Inch Pieces
- 2 ¾ Cups Vegetable Stock
- 1 Cup Arborio Rice, Rinsed & Drained
- 1 Teaspoon Thyme, Dried
- 1 Cup Sugar Snap Peas, Trimmed & Rinsed
- Sea Salt & Black Pepper to Taste
- Pinch Red Pepper Flakes
- 2 Tablespoons Vegan Butter
- 2 Cups Baby Spinach, Fresh & Torn
- ½ Lemon, Juiced

Directions:
1. Press sauté and set it to low, and then add in your oil.
2. Once it's hot, cook your onion for two minutes, stirring often.
3. Add in the asparagus and garlic, cooking for another thirty seconds.
4. Add in the salt, pepper, red pepper flakes, thyme, stock and rice.
5. Stir well and then seal the lid.

6. Cook on high pressure for eight minutes.
7. Use a quick release, and then stir in your vegan butter, spinach, and lemon juice.
8. Stir and serve warm.

Leek & Mushroom Risotto

Preparation time: 10 minutes
Cooking time: 50 minutes
Servings: 4

Ingredients:
- 4 Tablespoons Vegan Butter, Divided
- 1 Leek, Sliced
- 12 Ounces Baby Bella Mushrooms, Sliced
- 1 Cup Arborio Rice, Rinsed & Drained
- 2 Cloves Garlic, Minced
- 2 ¾ Cup Vegetable Stock
- 1 Teaspoon Thyme
- ½ Lemon, Juiced
- Sea Salt & Black Pepper to Taste
- Parsley, Fresh & Chopped for Garnish

Directions:
1. Press sauté and then turn it to low.
2. Add two tablespoons of butter, and once it's melted add in your mushrooms and leek. Sauté for two minutes, and stir often.
3. Add in your garlic, cooking for thirty seconds.
4. Throw in the rice, cooking for one minute and stirring often to toast it.
5. Turn it off of sauté.
6. Stir in your salt, thyme and stock.
7. Close the lid, and cook on high pressure for eight minutes.
8. Use a quick release.

9. Add lemon juice and two tablespoons of vegan butter, and then season with salt and pepper.
10. Garnish with parsley before serving.

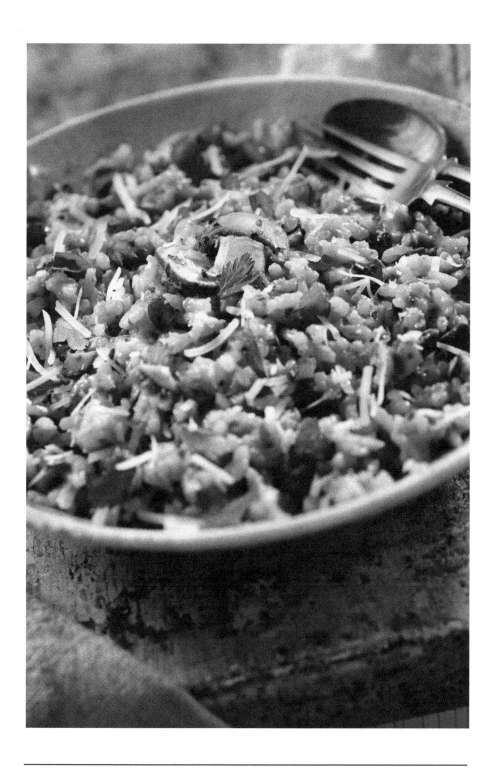

Cabbage Roll Bowls

Preparation time: 10 minutes
Cooking time: 40 minutes
Servings: 6

Ingredients:
Tempeh:
- 1 Tablespoon Olive Oil
- 8 Ounces Tempeh, Crumbled
- 2 Teaspoon Montreal Steak

Seasoning:
- 2 Cloves Garlic, Minced
- 2 Teaspoons Vegan Worcestershire Sauce
- 1 Bay Leaf
- ½ Onion, Diced Cabbage

Rolls:
- 1 Cup Basmati Rice, Rinsed & Drained
- 1 Cup Water
- 1 ½ Cups Vegetable Stock
- Sea Salt & Black Pepper to Taste
- 1 Head Cabbage, Sliced Thin
- 6 Ounces Tomato Paste
- ½ Teaspoon Paprika
- Pinch Cayenne Pepper
- ¼ Cup Parsley, Fresh & Chopped

Directions:
1. Select sauté and make sure it's set to low.

2. Once your instant pot is hot, add in your oil.
3. When your oil begins to shimmer, add in the tempeh with Montreal steak seasoning, garlic, bay leaf, Worcestershire shire sauce and onion.
4. Cook for four minutes, and then place it in a bowl.
5. Set the bowl to the side.
6. Clean your instant pot and then add in your water, salt and rice.
7. Lock the lid, and then cook on high pressure for eight minutes with the lid sealed.
8. Allow for a natural pressure release for ten minutes before following with a quick release.
9. Fluff the rice, and add in the cabbage, tomato paste, stock, paprika, pepper and cayenne.
10. Press sauté and select low.
11. Cook for five minutes.
12. Your cabbage should soften, and then discard the bay leaf.
13. Stir in your parsley, and serve warm with tempeh.

Coconut Rice & Veggies

Preparation time: 10 minutes
Cooking time: 30 minutes
Servings: 4

Ingredients:
- 1 Cup Jasmine Rice, Rinsed & Drained
- 1 Cup Water
- 1 Cup Bok Choy, Chopped
- 1 Carrot, Sliced
- 1 Onion, Small & Deiced
- 1 Tablespoon Sesame Oil
- ½ Teaspoon Ground Ginger
- Sea Salt & Black Pepper to Taste
- 1 Cup Sugar Snap Peas, Rinsed & Trimmed
- 8 Ounces Water Chestnuts, Canned, Sliced & Drained
- 2 Cloves Garlic, Minced
- 8 Ounces White Button Mushrooms, Sliced
- 14 Ounces Coconut Milk, Canned & Lite
- 1 Teaspoon Chinese Five Spice
- 1 Teaspoon Soy Sauce

Directions:
1. Combine your water, salt, ginger and rice.
2. Lock the lid and cook on high pressure for four minutes.
3. Use a natural pressure release for five minutes before following with a quick release.

4. Fluff the rice, and then place it in a bowl.
5. Set the rice to the side.
6. Press sauté and select low, and then add in your oil.
7. Once it's hot add in the carrot, bok choy, snap peas, onion, garlic, mushrooms and water chestnuts.
8. Cook for three minutes.
9. Stir in the five-spice powder, soy sauce, coconut milk and cooked rice.
10. Allow it to simmer for six minutes and serve warm.
11. The coconut milk should be reduced.

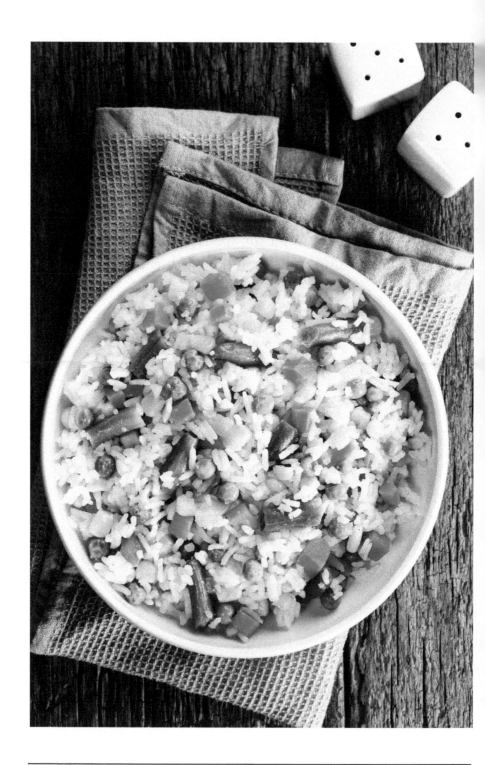

Quinoa & Butternut Chili

Preparation time: 10 minutes
Cooking time: 40 minutes
Servings: 4

Ingredients:
- 2 Tablespoons Olive Oil
- 2 Carrots, Sliced
- 1 Red Bell Pepper, Diced
- 1 Sweet Onion, Diced
- 1 Jalapeno Pepper, Diced
- 2 Cloves Garlic, Minced
- 1 Butternut Squash, Peeled & Cubed
- 14 Ounces Diced Tomatoes, Canned & With Juices
- 1 Cup Quinoa, Rinsed
- 1 Bay Leaf
- 1 Teaspoon Cumin
- 2 ½ Cups Vegetable Stock
- Sea Salt & Black Pepper to Taste
- ½ Teaspoon Chili Powder
- ½ Teaspoon Sweet Paprika
- 1 Teaspoon Cumin
- 1 Tablespoon Lemon Juice, Fresh

Directions:
1. Press sauté, and then add in your oil.
2. Once your oil is hot add in the jalapeno, bell pepper, carrots and onion.

3. Cook for three minutes, and stir often.
4. Turn it off of sauté, and then add in your garlic.
5. Stir and cook for thirty seconds.
6. Add your tomatoes, quinoa, stock bay leaf, squash, cumin, salt, paprika, chili powder and pepper.
7. Seal the lid, and cook on high pressure for eight minutes.
8. Use a natural pressure release for ten minutes, and then use a quick release.
9. Discard the bay leaf before stirring in your lemon juice.
10. Season with salt and pepper if desired.
11. If it is too liquid, press sauté and cook for two minutes more.

Beans, Grains and Dinner

Lentil and Chickpea Salad

Preparation time: 10 minutes
Cooking time: 0 minute
Servings: 4

Ingredients:
For the Lemon Dressing:
- ¼ cup lemon juice
- 2 tablespoons olive oil
- 1 teaspoon Dijon mustard
- 1 teaspoon honey or maple syrup
- ½ teaspoon minced garlic
- ¼ teaspoon of sea salt
- ¼ teaspoon ground black pepper

For the Salad:
- 2 cups French green lentils, cooked
- 1 ½ cups cooked chickpeas
- 1 medium avocado, pitted, sliced
- 1 big bunch of radishes, chopped
- ¼ cup chopped mint and dill
- Crumbled vegan feta cheese as needed

Directions:
1. Prepare the dressing and for this, place all of its ingredients in a bowl and whisk until combined.

2. Take a large bowl, place all the ingredients for the salad in it, drizzle with the dressing and toss until combined. Serve straight away.

Roasted Carrots with Farro, and Chickpeas

Preparation time: 10 minutes
Cooking time: 35 minutes
Servings: 4

Ingredients:
For the Chickpeas and Farro:
- 1 cup farro, cooked
- 1 ½ cups cooked chickpeas
- ½ teaspoon minced garlic
- 1 teaspoon lemon juice
- ½ teaspoon salt
- 1 teaspoon olive oil

For the Roasted Carrots:
- 1 pound heirloom carrots, scrubbed
- ½ teaspoon ground black pepper
- ¼ teaspoon ground cumin
- 1 teaspoon salt
- 1 tablespoon olive oil

For the Spiced Pepitas:
- 3 tablespoons green pumpkin seeds
- 1/8 teaspoon salt
- 1/8 teaspoon red chili powder
- 1/8 teaspoon cumin
- ½ teaspoon olive oil

For the Crème Fraiche:
- 1 tablespoon chopped parsley

- 1/3 cup vegan crème fraîche
- ¼ teaspoon ground black pepper
- 1/3 teaspoon salt
- 2 teaspoons water

For the Garnish:
- 1 more tablespoon chopped parsley

Directions:
1. Prepare chickpeas and farro and for this, place all of its ingredients in a bowl and toss until combined.
2. Prepare the carrots and for this, arrange them on a baking sheet lined with parchment paper, drizzle with oil, sprinkle with the seasoning, toss until coated, and bake for 35 minutes until roasted and fork-tender, turning halfway.
3. Meanwhile, prepare pepitas and for this, take a skillet pan, place it over medium heat, add oil and when hot, add remaining ingredients in it and cook for 3 minutes until seeds are golden on the edges, set aside, and let it cool.
4. Prepare the crème Fraiche and for this, place all its ingredients in a bowl and whisk until combined.
5. Top chickpeas and farro with carrots, drizzle with crème Fraiche, sprinkle with pepitas and parsley and then serve.

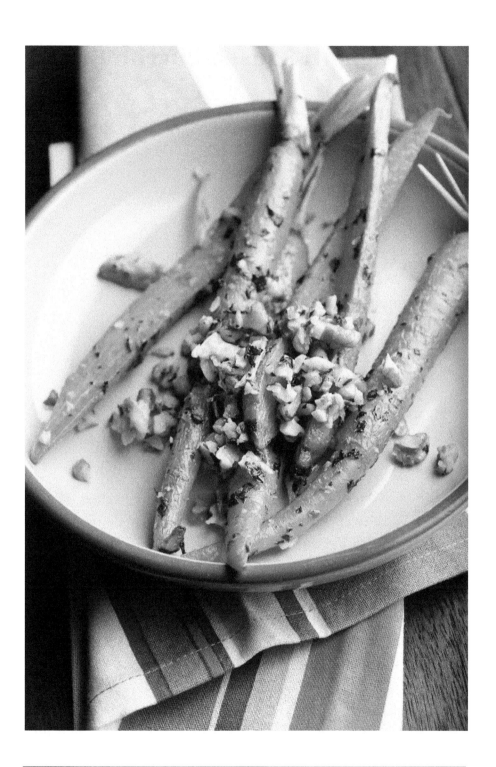

Spaghetti Squash Burrito Bowls

Preparation time: 10 minutes
Cooking time: 60 minutes
Servings: 4

Ingredients:
For the Spaghetti Squash:

- 2 medium spaghetti squash , halved, deseeded
- 2 tablespoons olive oil 1 teaspoon salt
- ½ teaspoon ground black pepper

For the Slaw:

- 1/3 cup chopped green onions
- 2 cups chopped purple cabbage
- 1/3 cup chopped cilantro
- 15 ounces cooked black beans
- 1 medium red bell pepper, cored, chopped
- ¼ teaspoon salt
- 1 teaspoon olive oil
- 2 tablespoons lime juice

For the Salsa Verde:

- 1 avocado, pitted, diced
- ½ teaspoon minced garlic
- ¾ cup salsa verde
- 1/3 cup cilantro
- 1 tablespoon lime juice

Directions:

1. Prepare the squash and for this, place squash halves on a baking sheet lined with parchment paper, rub

them with oil, season with salt and black pepper and bake for 60 minutes until roasted and fork-tender.
2. Meanwhile, place the slaw and for this, place all of its ingredients in a bowl and toss until combined.
3. Prepare the salsa, and for this, place all of its ingredients in a food processor and pulse until smooth.
4. When squash has baked, fluff its flesh with a fork, then top with slaw and salsa and serve.

Spanish Rice

Preparation time: 5 minutes
Cooking time: 40 minutes
Servings: 4

Ingredients:
- 1/2 of medium green bell pepper, chopped
- 1 medium white onion, peeled, chopped
- 10 ounces diced tomatoes with green chilies
- 1 teaspoon salt
- 2 teaspoons red chili powder
- 1 cup white rice
- 2 tablespoons olive oil
- 2 cups of water

Directions:
1. Take a large skillet pan, place it over medium heat, add oil and when hot, add onion, pepper, and rice, and cook for 10 minutes.
2. Then add remaining ingredients, stir until mixed, bring the mixture to a boil, then simmer over medium-low heat for 30 minutes until cooked and most of the liquid has absorbed.
3. Serve straight away.

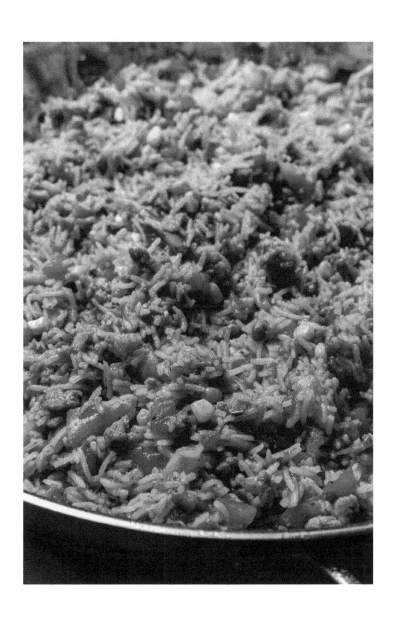

Black Beans and Rice

Preparation time: 10 minutes
Cooking time: 30 minutes
Servings: 4

Ingredients:
- 3/4 cup white rice
- 1 medium white onion, peeled, chopped
- 3 1/2 cups cooked black beans
- 1 teaspoon minced garlic
- 1/4 teaspoon cayenne pepper
- 1 teaspoon ground cumin
- 1 teaspoon olive oil
- 1 1/2 cups vegetable broth

Directions:
1. Take a large pot over medium-high heat, add oil and when hot, add onion and garlic and cook for 4 minutes until saute.
2. Then stir in rice, cook for 2 minutes, pour in the broth, bring it to a boil, switch heat to the low level and cook for 20 minutes until tender.
3. Stir in remaining ingredients, cook for 2 minutes, and then serve straight away.

Lentils and Rice with Fried Onions

Preparation time: 5 minutes
Cooking time: 7 minutes
Servings: 4

Ingredients:
- 3/4 cup long-grain white rice, cooked
- 1 large white onion, peeled, sliced
- 1 1/3 cups green lentils, cooked
- ½ teaspoon salt
- 1/4 cup vegan sour cream
- ¼ teaspoon ground black pepper
- 6 tablespoons olive oil

Directions:
1. Take a large skillet pan, place it over medium heat, add oil and when hot, add onions, and cook for 10 minutes until browned, set aside until required.
2. Take a saucepan, place it over medium heat, grease it with oil, add lentils and beans and cook for 3 minutes until warmed.
3. Season with salt and black pepper, cook for 2 minutes, then stir in half of the browned onions, and top with cream and remaining onions.
4. Serve straight away.

Mexican Stuffed Peppers

Preparation time: 10 minutes
Cooking time: 40 minutes
Servings: 4

Ingredients:
- 2 cups cooked rice
- 1/2 cup chopped onion
- 15 ounces cooked black beans
- 4 large green bell peppers, destemmed, cored
- 1 tablespoon olive oil
- 1 tablespoon salt
- 14.5 ounce diced tomatoes
- 1/2 teaspoon ground cumin
- 1 teaspoon garlic salt
- 1 teaspoon red chili powder
- 1/2 teaspoon salt
- 2 cups shredded vegan Mexican cheese blend

Directions:
1. Boil the bell peppers in salty water for 5 minutes until softened and then set aside until required.
2. Heat oil over medium heat in a skillet pan, then add onion and cook for 10 minutes until softened.
3. Transfer the onion mixture in a bowl, add remaining ingredients, reserving ½ cup cheese blended, stir until mixed, and then fill this mixture into the boiled peppers.

4. Arrange the peppers in the square baking dish, sprinkle them with remaining cheese and bake for 30 minutes at 350 degrees F.
5. Serve straight away.

Mushroom Risotto

Preparation time: 10 minutes
Cooking time: 35 minutes
Servings: 4

Ingredients:
- 1 cup of rice
- 3 small white onions, peeled, chopped
- 1 teaspoon minced celery
- 1 ½ cups sliced mushrooms
- ½ teaspoon minced garlic
- 1 teaspoon minced parsley
- ½ teaspoon salt
- ¼ teaspoon ground black pepper
- 1 tablespoon olive oil
- 1 teaspoon vegan butter
- ¼ cup vegan cashew cream
- 1 cup grated vegan Parmesan cheese
- 1 cup of coconut milk
- 5 cups vegetable stock

Directions:
1. Take a large skillet pan, place it over medium-high heat, add oil and when hot, add onion and garlic, and cook for 5 minutes.
2. Transfer to a plate, add celery and parsley into the pan, stir in salt and black pepper, and cook for 3 minutes.

3. Then switch heat to medium-low level, stir in mushrooms, cook for 5 minutes, then pour in cream and milk, stir in rice until combined, and bring the mixture to simmer.
4. Pour in vegetable stock, one cup at a time until it has absorbed and, when done, stir in cheese and butter.
5. Serve straight away.

Barley Bake

Preparation time: 10 minutes
Cooking time: 98 minutes
Servings: 6

Ingredients:
- 1 cup pearl barley
- 1 medium white onion, peeled, diced
- 2 green onions, sliced
- 1/2 cup sliced mushrooms
- 1/8 teaspoon ground black pepper
- 1/4 teaspoon salt
- 1/2 cup chopped parsley
- 1/2 cup pine nuts
- 1/4 cup vegan butter
- 29 ounces vegetable broth

Directions:
1. Place a skillet pan over medium-high heat, add butter and when it melts, stir in onion and barley, add nuts and cook for 5 minutes until light brown.
2. Add mushrooms, green onions and parsley, sprinkle with salt and black pepper, cook for 1 minute and then transfer the mixture into a casserole dish.
3. Pour in broth, stir until mixed and bake for 90 minutes until barley is tender and has absorbed all the liquid.
4. Serve straight away

Mushroom, Lentil, and Barley Stew

Preparation time: 10 minutes
Cooking time: 6 hours
Servings: 8

Ingredients:
- 3/4 cup pearl barley
- 2 cups sliced button mushrooms
- 3/4 cup dry lentils
- 1 ounce dried shiitake mushrooms
- 2 teaspoons minced garlic
- 1/4 cup dried onion flakes
- 2 teaspoons ground black pepper
- 1 teaspoon dried basil
- 2 ½ teaspoons salt
- 2 teaspoons dried savory
- 3 bay leaves
- 2 quarts vegetable broth

Directions:
1. Switch on the slow cooker, place all the ingredients in it, and stir until combined.
2. Shut with lid and cook the stew for 6 hours at a high heat until cooked.
3. Serve straight away.

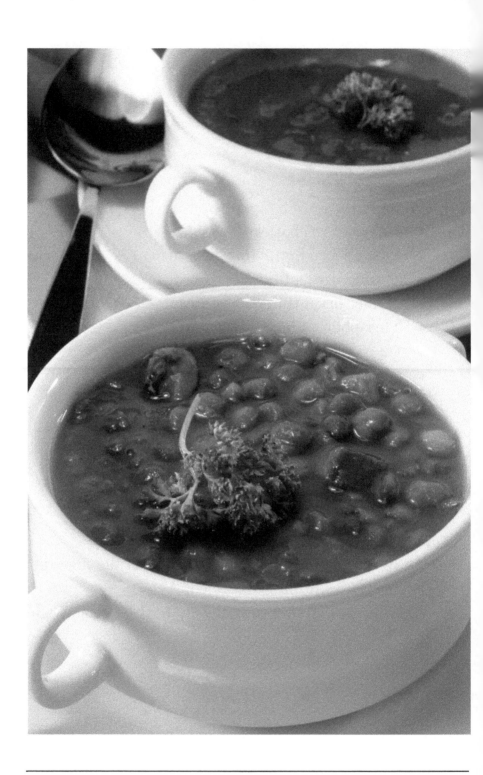

Black Beans, Corn, and Yellow Rice

Preparation time: 10 minutes
Cooking time: 25 minutes
Servings: 8

Ingredients:
- 8 ounces yellow rice mix
- 15.25 ounces cooked kernel corn
- 1 1/4 cups water
- 15 ounces cooked black beans
- 1 teaspoon ground cumin
- 2 teaspoons lime juice
- 2 tablespoons olive oil

Directions:
1. Place a saucepan over high heat, add oil, water, and rice, bring the mixture to a bowl, and then switch heat to medium-low level.
2. Simmer for 25 minutes until rice is tender and all the liquid has been absorbed and then transfer the rice to a large bowl.
3. Add remaining ingredients into the rice, stir until mixed and serve straight away.

Cuban Beans and Rice

Preparation time: 10 minutes
Cooking time: 55 minutes
Servings: 6

Ingredients:
- 1 cup uncooked white rice
- 1 green bell pepper, cored, chopped
- 15.25 ounces cooked kidney beans
- 1 cup chopped white onion
- 4 tablespoons tomato paste
- 1 teaspoon minced garlic
- 1 teaspoon salt
- 1 tablespoon olive oil
- 2 ½ cups vegetable broth

Directions:
1. Take a saucepan, place it over medium heat, add oil and when hot, add onion, garlic and bell pepper and cook for 5 minutes until tender.
2. Then stir in salt and tomatoes, switch heat to the low level and cook for 2 minutes.
3. Then stir in rice and beans, pour in the broth, stir until mixed and cook for 45 minutes until rice has absorbed all the liquid.
4. Serve straight away.

Pecan Rice

Preparation time: 5 minutes
Cooking time: 10 minutes
Servings: 4

Ingredients:
- 1/4 cup chopped white onion
- 1/4 teaspoon ground ginger
- 1/2 cup chopped pecans
- 1/4 teaspoon salt
- 2 tablespoons minced parsley
- 1/4 teaspoon ground black pepper
- 1/4 teaspoon dried basil
- 2 tablespoons vegan margarine
- 1 cup brown rice, cooked

Directions:
1. Take a skillet pan, place it over medium heat, add margarine and when it melts, add all the ingredients except for rice and stir until mixed.
2. Cook for 5 minutes, then stir in rice until combined and continue cooking for 2 minutes.
3. Serve straight away

Snacks and Sides

Zucchini Hummus

Preparation time: 5 minutes
Cooking time: 0 minute
Servings: 8

Ingredients:
- 1 cup diced zucchini
- 1/2 teaspoon sea salt
- 1 teaspoon minced garlic
- 2 teaspoons ground cumin
- 3 tablespoons lemon juice
- 1/3 cup tahini

Directions:
1. Place all the ingredients in a food processor and pulse for 2 minutes until smooth.
2. Tip the hummus in a bowl, drizzle with oil and serve.

Carrot and Sweet Potato Fritters

Preparation time: 10 minutes
Cooking time: 8 minutes
Servings: 10

Ingredients:
- 1/3 cup quinoa flour
- 1 ½ cups shredded sweet potato
- 1 cup grated carrot
- 1/3 teaspoon ground black pepper
- 2/3 teaspoon salt
- 2 teaspoons curry powder
- 2 flax eggs
- 2 tablespoons coconut oil

Directions:
1. Place all the ingredients in a bowl, except for oil, stir well until combined and then shape the mixture into ten small patties.
2. Take a large pan, place it over medium-high heat, add oil and when it melts, add patties in it and cook for 3 minutes per side until browned.
3. Serve straight.

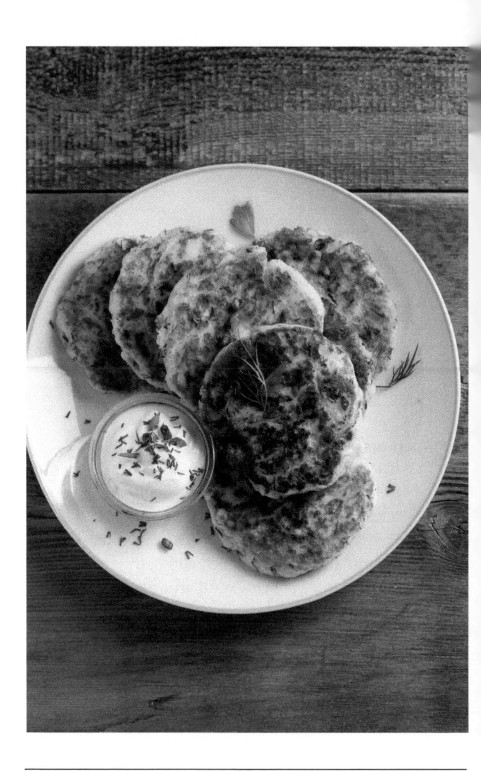

Tomato and Pesto Toast

Preparation time: 5 minutes
Cooking time: 0 minute
Servings: 4

Ingredients:
- 1 small tomato, sliced
- ¼ teaspoon ground black pepper
- 1 tablespoon vegan pesto
- 2 tablespoons hummus
- 1 slice of whole-grain bread, toasted
- Hemp seeds as needed for garnishing

Directions:
1. Spread hummus on one side of the toast, top with tomato slices and then drizzle with pesto.
2. Sprinkle black pepper on the toast along with hemp seeds and then serve straight away

Apple and Honey Toast

Preparation time: 5 minutes
Cooking time: 0 minute
Servings: 4

Ingredients:
- ½ of a small apple, cored, sliced
- 1 slice of whole-grain bread, toasted
- 1 tablespoon honey
- 2 tablespoons hummus
- 1/8 teaspoon cinnamon

Directions:
1. Spread hummus on one side of the toast, top with apple slices and then drizzle with honey.
2. Sprinkle cinnamon on it and then serve straight away.

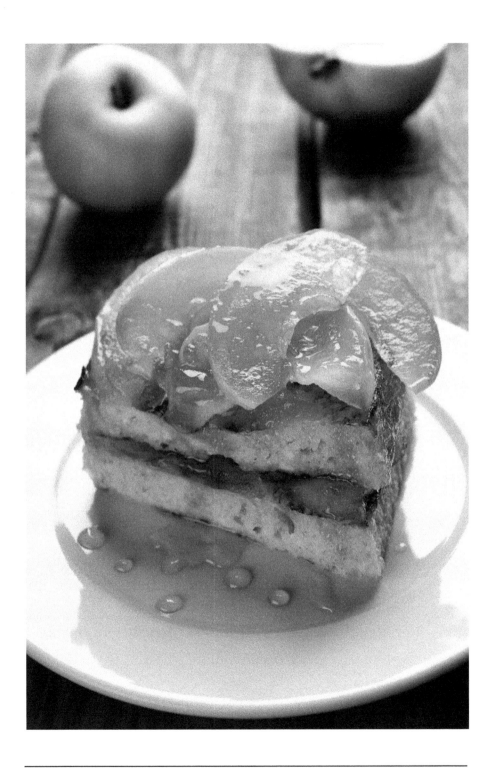

Zucchini Fritters

Preparation time: 10 minutes
Cooking time: 6 minutes
Servings: 12

Ingredients:
- 1/2 cup quinoa flour
- 3 1/2 cups shredded zucchini
- 1/2 cup chopped scallions
- 1/3 teaspoon ground black pepper
- 1 teaspoon salt
- 2 tablespoons coconut oil
- 2 flax eggs

Directions:
1. Squeeze moisture from the zucchini by wrapping it in a cheesecloth and then transfer it to a bowl.
2. Add remaining ingredients, except for oil, stir until combined and then shape the mixture into twelve patties.
3. Take a skillet pan, place it over medium-high heat, add oil and when hot, add patties and cook for 3 minutes per side until brown.
4. Serve the patties with your favorite vegan sauce.

Rosemary Beet Chips

Preparation time: 10 minutes
Cooking time: 20 minutes
Servings: 3

Ingredients:
- 3 large beets, scrubbed, thinly sliced
- 1/8 teaspoon ground black pepper
- ¼ teaspoon of sea salt
- 3 sprigs of rosemary, leaves chopped
- 4 tablespoons olive oil

Directions:
1. Spread beet slices in a single layer between two large baking sheets, brush the slices with oil, then season with spices and rosemary, toss until well coated, and bake for 20 minutes at 375 degrees F until crispy, turning halfway.
2. When done, let the chips cool for 10 minutes and then serve.

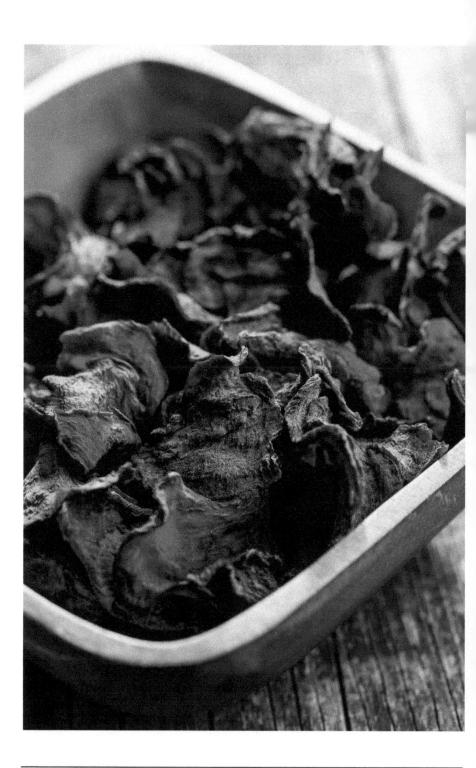

Spicy Roasted Chickpeas

Preparation time: 10 minutes
Cooking time: 20 minutes
Servings: 6

Ingredients:
- 30 ounces cooked chickpeas
- ½ teaspoon salt
- 2 teaspoons mustard powder
- ½ teaspoon cayenne pepper
- 2 tablespoons olive oil

Directions:
1. Place all the ingredients in a bowl and stir until well coated and then spread the chickpeas in an even layer on a baking sheet greased with oil.
2. Bake the chickpeas for 20 minutes at 400 degrees F until golden brown and crispy and then serve straight away.

Red Salsa

Preparation time: 10 minutes
Cooking time: 0 minute
Servings: 8

Ingredients:
- 30 ounces diced fire-roasted tomatoes
- 4 tablespoons diced green chilies
- 1 medium jalapeño pepper, deseeded
- 1/2 cup chopped green onion
- 1 cup chopped cilantro
- 1 teaspoon minced garlic
- ½ teaspoon of sea salt
- 1 teaspoon ground cumin
- ¼ teaspoon stevia
- 3 tablespoons lime juice

Directions:
1. Place all the ingredients in a food processor and process for 2 minutes until smooth.
2. Tip the salsa in a bowl, taste to adjust seasoning and then serve.

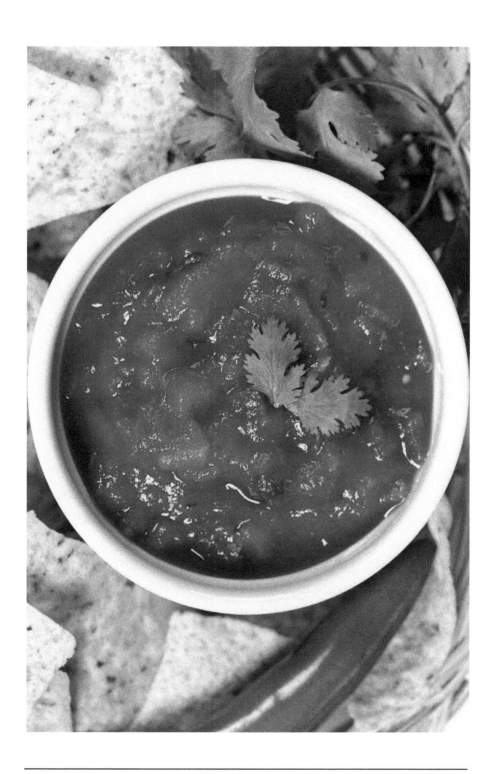

Hummus Quesadillas

Preparation time: 5 minutes
Cooking time: 15 minutes
Servings: 1

Ingredients:
- 1 tortilla, whole wheat
- 1/4 cup diced roasted red peppers
- 1 cup baby spinach
- 1/3 teaspoon minced garlic
- ¼ teaspoon salt
- ¼ teaspoon ground black pepper
- 1/4 teaspoon olive oil
- 1/4 cup hummus Oil as needed

Directions:
1. Place a large pan over medium heat, add oil and when hot, add red peppers and garlic, season with salt and black pepper and cook for 3 minutes until sauté.
2. Then stir in spinach, cook for 1 minute, remove the pan from heat and transfer the mixture in a bowl.
3. Prepare quesadilla and for this, spread hummus on one half of the tortilla, then spread spinach mixture on it, cover the filling with the other half of the tortilla and cook in a pan for 3 minutes per side until browned.
4. When done, cut the quesadilla into wedges and serve.

Avocado Tomato Bruschetta

Preparation time: 10 minutes
Cooking time: 0 minute
Servings: 4

Ingredients:
- 3 slices of whole-grain bread
- 6 chopped cherry tomatoes
- ½ of sliced avocado
- ½ teaspoon minced garlic
- ½ teaspoon ground black pepper
- 2 tablespoons chopped basil
- ½ teaspoon of sea salt
- 1 teaspoon balsamic vinegar

Directions:
1. Place tomatoes in a bowl, and then stir in vinegar until mixed.
2. Top bread slices with avocado slices, then top evenly with tomato mixture, garlic and basil, and season with salt and black pepper.
3. Serve straight

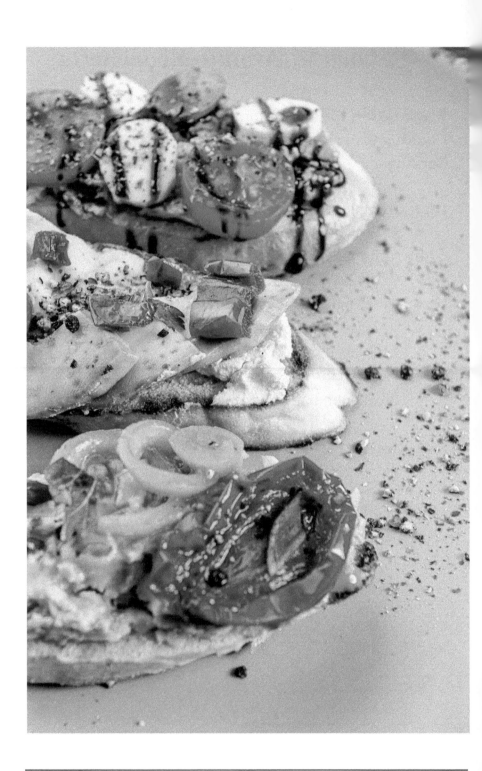

Salted Almonds

Preparation time: 5 minutes
Cooking time: 20 minutes
Servings: 4

Ingredients:
- 2 cups almonds
- 4 tablespoons salt
- 1 cup boiling water

Directions:
1. Stir the salt into the boiling water in a pan, then add almonds in it and let them soak for 20 minutes.
2. Then drain the almonds, spread them in an even layer on a baking sheet lined with baking paper and sprinkle with salt.
3. Roast the almonds for 20 minutes at 300 degrees F, then cool them for 10 minutes and serve.

Honey-Almond Popcorn

Preparation time: 5 minutes
Cooking time: 10 minutes
Servings: 4

Ingredients:
- 1/2 cup popcorn kernels
- 2 tablespoons honey
- 1/2 teaspoon sea salt
- 2 tablespoons coconut sugar
- 1 cup roasted almonds
- 1/4 cup walnut oil

Directions:
1. Take a pot, place it over medium-low heat, add oil and when it melts, add four kernels and wait until they sizzle.
2. Then add remaining kernel, toss until coated, sprinkle with sugar, drizzle with honey, shut the pot with the lid, and shake the kernels until popped completely, adding almonds halfway.
3. Once all the kernels have popped, season them with salt and serve straight away.

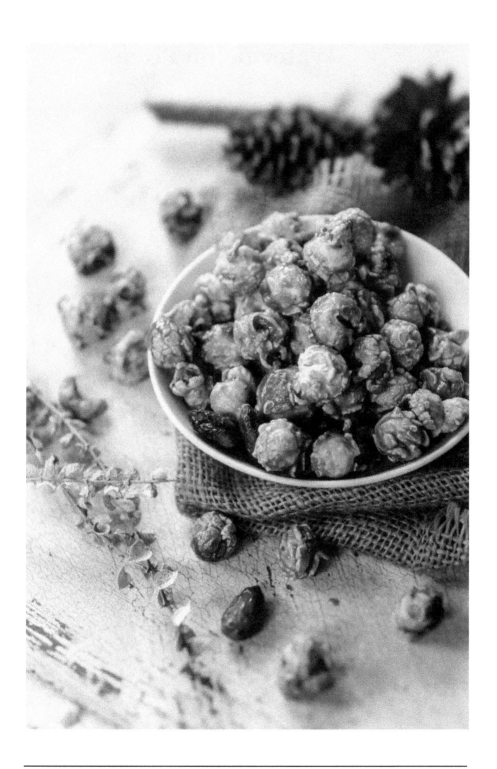

Watermelon Pizza

Preparation time: 10 minutes
Cooking time: 0 minute
Servings: 10

Ingredients:
- 1/2 cup strawberries, halved
- 1/2 cup blueberries
- 1 watermelon
- 1/2 cup raspberries
- 1 cup of coconut yogurt
- 1/2 cup pomegranate seeds
- 1/2 cup cherries Maple syrup as needed

Directions:
1. Cut watermelon into 3-inch thick slices, then spread yogurt on one side, leaving some space in the edges and then top evenly with fruits and drizzle with maple syrup.
2. Cut the watermelon into wedges and then serve.

Desserts

Chocolate Avocado Ice Cream

Preparation time: 1 hour and 10 minutes
Cooking time: 0 minute
Servings: 2

Ingredients:
- 4.5 ounces avocado, peeled, pitted
- 1/2 cup cocoa powder, unsweetened
- 1 tablespoon vanilla extract, unsweetened
- 1/2 cup and 2 tablespoons maple syrup
- 13.5 ounces coconut milk, unsweetened
- 1/2 cup water

Directions:
1. Add avocado in a food processor along with milk and then pulse for 2 minutes until smooth.
2. Add remaining ingredients, blend until mixed, and then tip the pudding in a freezer-proof container.
3. Place the container in a freezer and chill for 4 hours until firm, whisking every 20 minutes after 1 hour.
4. Serve straight away.

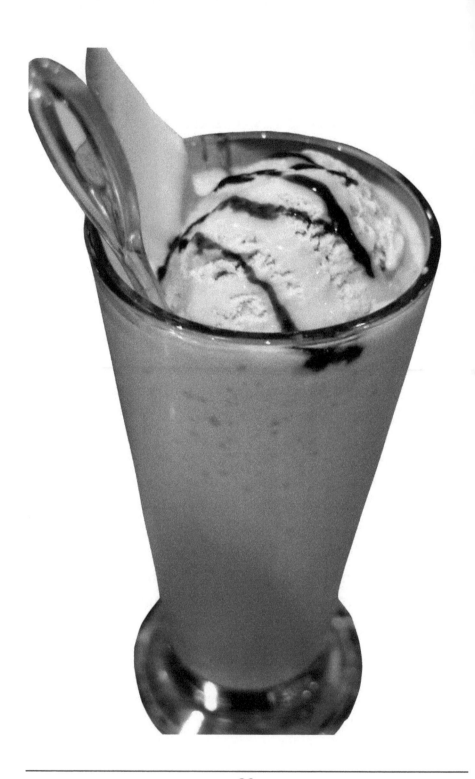

Mango Coconut Chia Pudding

Preparation time: 2 hours and 5 minutes
Cooking time: 0 minute
Servings: 1

Ingredients:
- 1 medium mango, peeled, cubed
- 1/4 cup chia seeds
- 2 tablespoons coconut flakes
- 1 cup coconut milk, unsweetened
- 1 1/2 teaspoons maple syrup

Directions:
1. Take a bowl, place chia seeds in it, whisk in milk until combined, and then stir in maple syrup.
2. Cover the bowl with a plastic wrap; it should touch the pudding mixture and refrigerate for 2 hours until the pudding has set.
3. Then puree mango until smooth, top it evenly over pudding, sprinkle with coconut flakes and serve.

Strawberry Coconut Ice Cream

Preparation time: 5 minutes
Cooking time: 0 minute
Servings: 4

Ingredients:
- 4 cups frozen strawberries
- 1 vanilla bean, seeded
- 28 ounces coconut cream
- 1/2 cup maple syrup

Directions:
1. Place cream in a food processor and pulse for 1 minute until soft peaks come together.
2. Then tip the cream in a bowl, add remaining ingredients in the blender and blend until a thick mixture comes together.
3. Add the mixture into the cream, fold until combined, and then transfer ice cream into a freezer-safe bowl and freeze for 4 hours until firm, whisking every 20 minutes after 1 hour.
4. Serve straight away

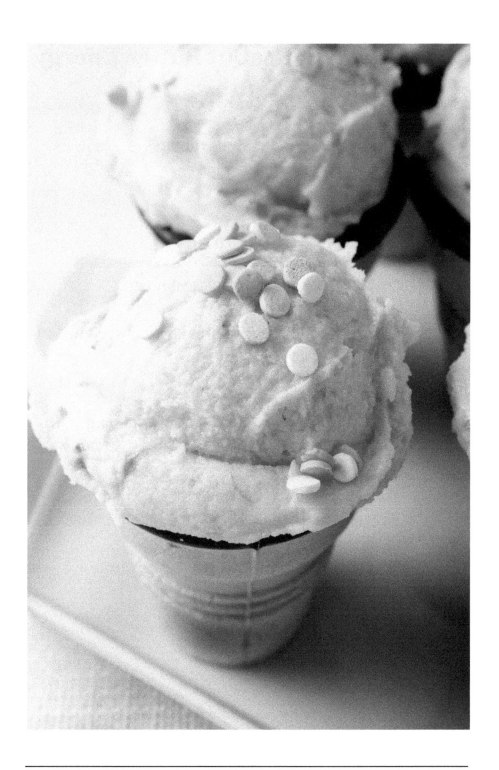

Chocolate Peanut Butter Energy Bites

Preparation time: 1 hour and 5 minutes
Cooking time: 0 minute
Servings: 4

Ingredients:
- 1/2 cup oats, old-fashioned
- 1/3 cup cocoa powder, unsweetened
- 1 cup dates, chopped
- 1/2 cup shredded coconut flakes, unsweetened
- 1/2 cup peanut butter

Directions:
1. Place oats in a food processor along with dates and pulse for 1 minute until the paste starts to come together.
2. Then add remaining ingredients, and blend until incorporated and a very thick mixture comes together.
3. Shape the mixture into balls, refrigerate for 1 hour until set and then serve.

Rainbow Fruit Salad

Preparation time: 10 minutes
Cooking time: 0 minute
Servings: 4

Ingredients:
For the Fruit Salad:
- 1 pound strawberries, hulled, sliced
- 1 cup kiwis, halved, cubed
- 1 1/4 cups blueberries
- 1 1/3 cups blackberries
- 1 cup pineapple chunks

For the Maple Lime Dressing:
- 2 teaspoons lime zest
- 1/4 cup maple syrup
- 1 tablespoon lime juice

Directions:
1. Prepare the salad, and for this, take a bowl, place all its ingredients and toss until mixed.
2. Prepare the dressing, and for this, take a small bowl, place all its ingredients and whisk well.
3. Drizzle the dressing over salad, toss until coated and serve.

Dark Chocolate Bars

Preparation time: 1 hour and 10 minutes
Cooking time: 2 minutes
Servings: 12

Ingredients:
- 1 cup cocoa powder, unsweetened
- 3 Tablespoons cacao nibs
- 1/8 teaspoon sea salt
- 2 Tablespoons maple syrup
- 1 1/4 cup chopped cocoa butter
- 1/2 teaspoons vanilla extract, unsweetened
- 2 Tablespoons coconut oil

Directions:
1. Take a heatproof bowl, add butter, oil, stir, and microwave for 90 to 120 seconds until it melts, stirring every 30 seconds.
2. Sift cocoa powder over melted butter mixture, whisk well until combined, and then stir in maple syrup, vanilla, and salt until mixed.
3. Distribute the mixture evenly between twelve mini cupcake liners, top with cacao nibs, and freeze for 1 hour until set.
4. Serve straight away.

Chocolate and Avocado Truffles

Preparation time: 1 hour and 10 minutes
Cooking time: 1 minute
Servings: 18

Ingredients:
- 1 medium avocado, ripe
- 2 tablespoons cocoa powder
- 10 ounces of dark chocolate chips

Directions:
1. Scoop out the flesh from the avocado, place it in a bowl, then mash with a fork until smooth, and stir in 1/2 cup chocolate chips.
2. Place remaining chocolate chips in a heatproof bowl and microwave for 1 minute until chocolate has melted, stirring halfway.
3. Add melted chocolate into avocado mixture, stir well until blended, and then refrigerate for 1 hour.
4. Then shape the mixture into balls, 1 tablespoon of mixture per ball, and roll in cocoa powder until covered.
5. Serve straight away.

Dark Chocolate Raspberry Ice Cream

Preparation time: 5 minutes
Cooking time: 0 minute
Servings: 2

Ingredients:
- 2 frozen bananas, sliced
- ¼ cup fresh raspberries
- 2 tablespoons cocoa powder, unsweetened
- 2 tablespoons raspberry jelly

Directions:
1. Place all the ingredients in a food processor, except for berries and pulse for 2 minutes until smooth.
2. Distribute the ice cream mixture between two bowls, stir in berries until combined, and then serve immediately

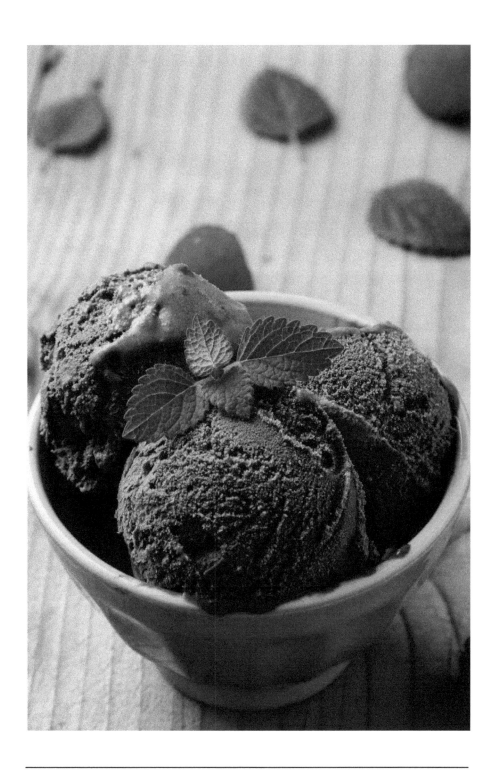

Peanut Butter and Honey Ice Cream

Preparation time: 5 minutes
Cooking time: 0 minute
Servings: 2

Ingredients:
- 2½ tablespoons peanut butter
- 2 bananas frouncesen, sliced
- 1½ tablespoons honey

Directions:
1. Place all the ingredients in a food processor and pulse for 2 minutes until smooth.
2. Distribute the ice cream mixture between two bowls and then serve immediately.

Chocolate Pudding

Preparation time: 5 minutes
Cooking time: 0 minute
Servings: 4

Ingredients:
- 3/4 cup cocoa powder
- 12 ounces tofu, silken
- 1/3 cup almond milk, unsweetened
- 1/2 cup sugar Whipped cream for topping

Directions:
1. Place all the ingredients in a food processor and pulse for 2 minutes until smooth.
2. Distribute the pudding between four bowls, refrigerate for 15 minutes, then top with whipped topping and serve immediately.

Almond Butter Cookies

Preparation time: 35 minutes
Cooking time: 5 minutes
Servings: 13

Ingredients:
- 1/4 cup sesame seeds
- 1 cup rolled oats
- 3 Tablespoons sunflower seeds, roasted, unsalted
- 1/8 teaspoon sea salt
- 1 1/2 Tablespoons coconut flour
- 1/2 cup coconut sugar
- 1/2 teaspoons vanilla extract, unsweetened
- 3 Tablespoons coconut oil
- 2 Tablespoons almond milk, unsweetened
- 1/3 cup almond butter, salted

Directions:
1. Take a saucepan, place it over medium heat, pour in milk, stir in sugar and oil and bring the mixture to a low boil.
2. Boil the mixture for 1 minute, then remove the pan from heat, and stir in remaining ingredients until incorporated and well combined.
3. Drop the prepared mixture onto a baking sheet lined with wax paper, about 13 cookies, and let the cookies stand for 25 minutes until firm and set.
4. Serve straight away.

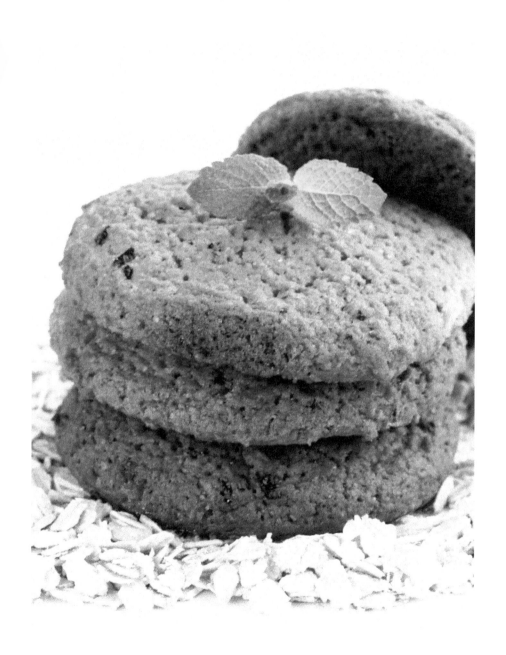

Coconut Cacao Bites

Preparation time: 1 hour and 10 minutes
Cooking time: 0 minute
Servings: 20

Ingredients:
- 1 1/2 cups almond flour
- 3 dates, pitted
- 1 1/2 cups shredded coconut, unsweetened
- 1/4 teaspoons ground cinnamon
- 2 Tablespoons flaxseed meal
- 1/16 teaspoon sea salt
- 2 Tablespoons vanilla protein powder
- 1/4 cup cacao powder
- 3 Tablespoons hemp seeds
- 1/3 cup tahini
- 4 Tablespoons coconut butter, melted

Directions:
1. Place all the ingredients in a food processor and pulse for 5 minutes until the thick paste comes together.
2. Drop the mixture in the form of balls on a baking sheet lined with parchment sheet, 2 tablespoons per ball and then freeze for 1 hour until firm to touch.
3. Serve straight away.

Chocolate Cookies

Preparation time: 40 minutes
Cooking time: 5 minutes
Servings: 4

Ingredients:
- 1/2 cup coconut oil
- 1 cup agave syrup
- 1/2 cup cocoa powder
- 1/2 teaspoon salt
- 2 cups peanuts, chopped
- 1 cup peanut butter
- 2 cups sunflower seeds

Directions:
1. Take a small saucepan, place it over medium heat, add the first three ingredients, and cook for 3 minutes until melted.
2. Boil the mixture for 1 minute, then remove the pan from heat and stir in salt and butter until smooth.
3. Fold in nuts and seeds until combined, then drop the mixture in the form of molds onto the baking sheet lined with wax paper and refrigerate for 30 minutes.
4. Serve straight away.

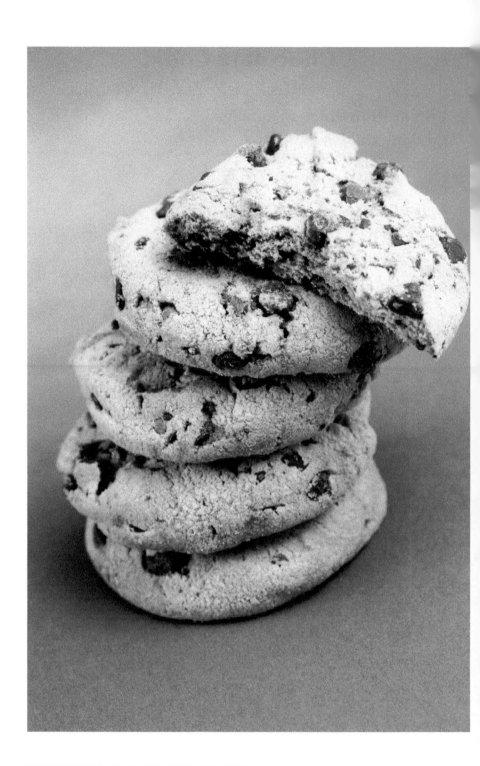

Notes

Lightning Source UK Ltd.
Milton Keynes UK
UKHW020814170621
385664UK00001B/180